Dukan

The Ultimate Dukan Diet Guide- How To

Lose Weight Fast With The Dukan Diet

Plan

(Dukan Diet Recipes For Beginners)

Dexter Erickson

TABLE OF CONTENTS

Chicken Kebabs

Ingredients:

Chicken breast, diced, 6 00 gm

1 fresh lemon juice

Saffron, 1/2 tsp

Black pepper, 1 tsp

Ginger, 1 tsp

Turmeric, 1 tsp

Garlic, crushed, 2 cloves

Paprika, 2 tsp

Instructions:

1. Add all ingredients to a shallow bowl and blend until properly combine.
2. Cover and let it chill in refrigerator for about 55 minutes.
3. Make kebabs in skewers.
4. Cook kebabs onto griddle pan onto high heat and until golden before you serve.

Salmon and Cream Cheese Wrap

Ingredients:

Chives, sliced, 2 tbsp

Oat bran, 4 tbsp

Black pepper

Cream cheese, low-fat, 2 tbsp

Greek yogurt, 4 tbsp

Smoked salmon, few slices

Fresh Fresh egg s, 2

Instructions:

1. Take a bowl; add all ingredients except chives and whisk well to form batter.
2. Now add chives to mixture.
3. Decant half the batter in a pan coated with oil and cook until both sides are golden.
4. Do the same for remaining batter.
5. Arrange pancakes in a serving dish and keep aside to cool for few minutes.
6. Press with cream and add salmon topping.
7. Season with pepper before you fold and serve.

Oat Bran Galette with Toffee Yogurt

Ingredients:

Toffee yogurt, low-fat, 2 small pot

Greek yogurt, 2 tbsp

Sweetener, 2 tsp

Fresh Fresh egg , 2

Oat bran, 2 tbsp

Instructions:

1. Take a bowl; add fresh Fresh egg , oat bran, sweetener as well as yogurt and combine.

2. Add half the mixture in a frying pan coated with oil and cook pancakes on medium high heat until golden.
3. Arrange onto platters; wrap it with lid and do the same with remaining mixture.
4. Serve alongside toffee yogurt.

Coffee Frappuccino

Ingredients:

Oat Bran:

Greek yogurt, 4 tbsp

Fresh egg whites, 2

Spices of choice

Oat bran, 4 tbsp

Filling:

Cream cheese, low-fat, 2 tbsp

Lean meat, cooked

Instructions:

1. In a bowl; add all ingredients together and whisk until form batter.
2. Add a bit of yogurt if batter is too thick; flavor with spices and favorite herbs.
3. Place half the mixture on frying pan coated with oil and cook until light brown.
4. Set aside.
5. Do the same for remaining mixture and arrange it on platters.

6. Halve galette and scatter cream on each sides.
7. Stuff cooked meat in there before you serve.

Homemade Yogurt

Ingredients:

Boiling water, 4 tsp

Yogurt, fat-free, 2 large tub

Jelly, sugar-free, 4 tsp

Instructions:

1. Take a bowl; add boiling water and whisk jelly properly until properly dissolved.
2. Keep it aside for about 4 minutes and to chill.
3. In a food processor; add jelly syrup as well as yogurt and process until smooth before you serve.

Oat bran porridge

Ingredients

- 2 egg, lightly beaten
- 2 -2 tbs finely chopped basil or mint
- Optional Salad to serve
- Salt and pepper to taste
- 2 onion, chopped
- mog minced beef
- 2 tablespoons plum sauce
- 2 garlic cloves, crushed
- 2 tablespoons finely chopped rosemary
  2 tablespoon Worcestershire sauce

Instructions

1. Mix all ingredients then shape into patties and transfer to the microwave then microwave until golden brown on both sides. Drain on paper towel.

10

Fishcake

Ingredients

- 2 white fish fillet, chopped Chopped herbs, to taste
- 4 crabsticks, thinly sliced
- 6 tablespoons fat-free quark 4 eggs, separated
- 2 garlic clove, crushed
- 2 tablespoon corn flour

Instructions

1. Beat fresh egg whites until stiff. Blend in the other ingredients and bake at 2 80°C for 50 minutes.

Dessert

Chocolate Coffee Meringues

Ingredients

- 4 fresh egg whites
- 2 teaspoons of very strong coffee 6 tbsp of sweetener
- 2 teaspoons cocoa powder

Instructions

1. Preheat oven to 2 .6 0°C. Beat the fresh egg whites until stiff then blend the cocoa with sweetener and then spread over the fresh egg whites.

2. Add in the coffee and beat for another 45 seconds.

3. Transfer into small mounds on a baking tray and microwave for 35 to 40 minutes.

12

Oat Bran Muffins

Ingredients

- 1 teaspoon sweetener
- 4 tablespoons fromage frais Lemon zest or cinnamon
- 8 tablespoons oat bran
- 4 eggs, separated

Instructions

1. Pre-heat oven to 2 80°C. Beat fresh egg whites until stiff then blend in the other ingredients.
2. Press in fresh egg whites then transfer into cases and bake for 20-45 minutes.

Prawn And Fresh egg Salad

Ingredients

- A few sprigs tarragon
- 600g lettuce 4 eggs
- 200 g cooked and shelled prawns
- 4 teaspoons cider vinegar
- 2 teaspoon olive oil

Instructions

1. Prepare vinaigrette with vinegar and oil, then season with salt and pepper.
2. Blend tarragon leaves prawns and lettuce in a bowl.
3. Dip the eggs in boiling water for six minutes until soft then remove shells and serve hot with prawns and dressed lettuce.

Salmon Escalopes

Ingredients

- 2 tablespoon mild mustard
- Finely chopped dill, to taste
- Steamed asparagus (optional)
- 2 chopped shallots
- 4 thick pieces of salmon
- 6 teaspoons fat-free fromage frais

Instructions

1. Place salmon in the freezer for a few minutes and then cut it into thin slices.
2. Gently fry these slices in a non-stick pan for 2 minute on both sides then set aside while warm.
3. Cook shallots until brown then add fromage frais and mustard and simmer for 10 minutes.

15

4. Put the salmon back into the pan and sprinkle dill and season with salt and pepper then cook until set and serve with asparagus.

Chocolate Pannacotta

Ingredients

- 2 fresh egg yolks
- 2 gelatine leaves
- 2 tablespoon protein powder
- 2 tablespoon of cocoa powder
- 6 tablespoons fat-free fromage frais
- 250 ml skimmed milk

Instructions

1. Soften the gelatine in a bowl with cold water then combine the cocoa powder, fresh egg yolks, and protein powder in another bowl and set aside. Boil milk in a small saucepan then pour in the fresh egg mixture and stir to mix.

2. Drain excess water from the gelatine and blend into the hot mixture until completely dissolved.

3. Let this cool, before adding the fromage frais.

Skim Milk And Muesli

Ingredients

- 2 fresh egg
- 6 tablespoons oat bran
- Almond essence
- 2 tablespoon liquid sweetener

Instructions

1. Preheat oven to 2 60°C. Blend all ingredients and place on baking-paper-lined tray. Bake for 45 minutes.
2. Wait until cool then crumble. Preserve in an airtight container.

Salmon Pancakes

Ingredients

- 4 slices smoked salmon
- 2 small jar salmon roe
- 2 oat bran pancakes
- bog fat-free quark
- 4 oog fat-free fromage frais

Instruction

1. Blend the roe, quark and fromage frais in a bowl and season.
2. Split this among pancakes and top with salmon.

Chicken Kebabs

*I*ngredients

- 250 g of fat-free plain yogurt
- 2 teaspoon garam masala
- ¹ tablespoon ground cumin
- 800g chunked chicken breasts
- 2 tablespoons finely chopped coriander
- Tzatziki, to serve
- 2 peeled garlic clove
- 2 onion, peeled
- 2 tablespoons lemon juice
- 250 g grated ginger
- 1 tablespoons ground coriander

Instructions

1. Purée garlic and onion in a blender. Blend in lemon juice, coriander, ginger, spices, and yogurt.

2. Add marinade to the chicken then chill for 2 hours.

3. Preheat the grill on high then place chicken on skewers and place on the grill. Leave to cook for 825 minutes and then serve with fat-free tzatziki.

Orange Yogurt Cake

Ingredients

- 2 teaspoons yeast
- 4 tablespoons corn flour
- 4 drops of vegetable oil
- 2 6 0 g fat-free natural yogurt
- 4 eggs
- 2 teaspoon orange extract
- 1 teaspoon artificial sweetener

Instructions

1. Preheat the oven to 2 80°C. Blend eggs with yogurt, and then add orange extract, sweetener, yeast, and corn flour.

2. Pour into a cake tin and bake for 50 minutes.

Dukan Oat Pancakes

Ingredients:

- 5 tbsp. bran, oat
- 5 tbsp. quark (cheese, fresh acid-set)
- 2 fresh Fresh egg , large

Instructions:

1.
   Pour oat bran in medium bowl.
2. Add fresh egg and quark. Mix ingredients well. Pour onto pre-greased non-stick pan.

3. Cook for two to three minutes per side. Serve.

Breakfast Cream Cheese Casserole

Ingredients:

- 2 cans of crescent rolls, reduced fat
- 2 pound of browned sausage
- 8 ounces of cream cheese, fat-free

Instructions:

1.

Spread 2 can crescent rolls on the bottom of a 2 4 x10 -inch pan. Pinch the seams.

Cover the spread rolls with cream cheese and sausage.

2. Spread other can crescent rolls on top of sausage and cream cheese mixture.

3. Bake using instructions on package. Serve.

4 – Oat Bran Dukan Porridge

Ingredients:

- 4 tbsp. of bran, oat
- 4 tbsp. of milk powder, skim
- 2 fresh egg whites from large fresh egg s
- 2 tbsp. of sugar substitute
- 25 1 fluid ounces of milk, skim

Instructions:

1.

   Mix all your ingr

2. edients except milk in breakfast sized bowl.

   Add milk slowly and stir till there are no

lumps.

3. Cook in microwave for a minute and a half on 8 6 0 power level. Stir well. Cook for a minute more on 66 0 power level.   Stir   again.

4. Cook at one-minute intervals on 66 0 till cooked   fully.   Serve.

Sausage Scramble with Jalapenos

Ingredients:

- 2 fresh Fresh egg s, large
- 4 large fresh egg whites
- 2 helpings of sausage, turkey
- 1 sliced onion, small

Instructions:

1.

Brown onion and sausage in non-stick pan.

Add the fresh egg s and combine. Serve.

2. 6 – Super Breakfast Smoothie

Ingredients:

- 2 pkt. of milk chocolate instant breakfast mix
- 2 cup of milk, fat-free
- 6 ounces of yogurt, strawberry
- 1 cup of strawberries, frozen, whole

Instructions:

1. Place all the ingredients in food processor.
2. Blend for a minute till smooth. Serve.

Chicken Meatballs

Ingredients:

- 2 lb. of chicken, ground
- 2 chopped onion, small
- 2 minced clove of garlic, small
- 2 fresh Fresh egg , large
- Spices: kosher salt, ground pepper and garlic powder
- 2 tbsp. of bran, oat
- 4 tbsp. of chopped dill or parsley

Instructions:

1.

Preheat oven to 480F. Mince garlic and onion.

33

Add all ingredients to large bowl. Mix them together well. Form the mixture into 30 to 25 balls and place on a pan.

2. Bake in the middle rack of 4 6 0F oven for 30-35 minutes, till juices are running clear.

Remove from oven and serve.

Dukan Lime-Kissed Shrimp

Ingredients:

- 2 dashes of salt, kosher
  - 1/3 tsp. of pepper, black, ground
  - 2 tbsp. of chopped onion

- Non-stick spray
  - 28 ready to cook shrimp, large
  - 1 juiced

- lime

Instructions:

Spray a skillet with non-stick spray. Heat it over med. heat. Add the ingredients. Cook till onions and shrimp   are   done.   Serve.

Zucchini Lasagna

Ingredients:

4   1 oz. of mozzarella cheese, light
- 2   tbsp. of tomato extract, pure
-     1   onion,   medium
-     2   garlic   clove
- As desired: oregano, chives, parsley, kosher salt and

2 lengthways-sliced zucchinis, medium
- 2 peeled, de-seeded tomatoes, ripe, large
- 8   ounces of ground beef, lean
- 4   1 oz. of turkey breast, smoked

ground   pepper

Instructions:

Grill each side of sliced zucchinis in non-stick pan. Set aside. 2. Sauté onion and garlic in pan on low heat. Add kosher salt, ground pepper and beef. Cook on low. 4 . Pour 2 1/3 fl. oz. of filtered water in food processor. Add chives, parsley and tomatoes (diced). Combine till smooth. 4. Add sauce to beef. Add tomato extract. Boil mixture for 2 2-30 minutes.

6 . Add some sauce to baking dish/pizza form for oven cooking. Form layers using zucchini, then turkey breast, then cheese and sauce. Repeat layers two times. Top with cheese and oregano. 6. Place in oven for 20-210 minutes. Then turn oven to off. Allow lasagna to sit for 2 2-30 minutes. Serve.

Dukan Chili

Ingredients:

- 5 lb. of chuck, ground
- 5 lb. of onions, chopped
- 2 cup of chopped bell pepper, green
- 2 chopped and de-seeded jalapeno
- 2 tbsp. of garlic, chopped
- 2 tbsp. of chili powder
- 2 tbsp. of Worcestershire sauce
- 5 tsp. of cumin, ground
- 2 tsp. of paprika, smoked
- 2 tsp. of salt, kosher
- 1 tsp. of pepper, ground
- 2 x 6-ounce can of tomato paste
- 2 x 2 4 1 ounce can of broth, beef
- 2 can of undrained tomatoes, diced
- 2 can of undrained kidney beans

- 2　can of undrained pinto beans
- 2　cup of cheddar cheese shreds

Instructions:

1. Cook the ground chuck, onions, bell peppers, garlic and jalapeno in large sized pan on med-high heat for 8-25 minutes.

2. Crumble beef as you cook. It should not be pink at all when you're done.

3. Stir the mixture occasionally and drain.

4. Add tomato paste, kosher salt, ground pepper, paprika, cumin and chili powder.

5. Cook for a couple minutes until they are fragrant.

6. Add in and stir the Worcestershire sauce, undrained tomatoes and beans.

7. Bring to boil and reduce heat. Cover and simmer for 40-50 minutes, while you occasionally stir the mixture. Serve with the cheese.

Cheese and Garlic Chicken Pocket

Ingredients:

- 2 breasts of chicken
- 4 tbsp. of fat-free cream cheese
- Garlic powder, as desired
- Salt, kosher, as desired

Instructions:

1.

Preheat oven to 480F. Slice chicken breasts in middle area. Create pockets. Don't slice completely through.

Sprinkle garlic powder and kosher salt as desired inside pockets created in step

43

Spread aluminum foil in roasting tray. It should be of sufficient size to put chicken breasts inside and wrap meat.

2. Place 5 to 10 tbsp. of cream cheese in pockets.

3. Add additional garlic powder, if desired.

4. Seal meat up using your fingers.

5. Sprinkle parsley over the top.

Cheesy Broccoli Casserole

Ingredients:

- 2 x 25 2 /2-ounce cans of cream of mushroom soup, condensed
- 2 cup of milk, 2%
- 1 tsp. of pepper, black, ground
- 2 lbs. of cooked to tender-crisp, well-drained florets of broccoli
- 2 cups of cheddar cheese shreds
- 2 x 6-oz. container of crispy fried onions

Instructions:

1.

Preheat the oven to 480F. Mix the

milk, pepper and soup in a large sized bowl.

 Add 2 cup fried onions, 2 cup of cheese and the broccoli. Toss and coat gently.

Spoon the mixture in 10 x2 4 " greased baking dish. Cover dish with aluminum foil.

Bake for 1 hour. Remove the foil and stir fully. Sprinkle on the rest of the fried onions and cheese. Leave uncovered and bake for 15-20 minutes, till onions become a golden brown and the cheese gets bubbly. Serve.

Chicken Marsala

Ingredients:

- 2 chicken breast
- 2 tbsp. of curry powder
- 4 tbsp. of garam masala (Middle Eastern spice mix)
- 2 tbsp. of garlic powder
- 2 handful of mushrooms
- 1/2 of 2 small onion, red
- 2 tbsp. of milk, skim

Instructions:

Butterfly-cut chicken thinly, so it cooks quicker. Add curry powder and garlic salt on each side of chicken. Use oven or grill to cook chicken till both sides are brown.

47

As chicken cooks, slice mushrooms and onions into pieces of 2 /2-inch or so. Add to sauté pan. As the mushrooms start shrinking, add milk. Turn heat down. Allow to simmer for about five more minutes. Place chicken on plates and spread the onion and mushroom mixture over the top. Serve.

Spinach Pie

Ingredients:

- 2 handful of basil leaves, chopped
- 2   handful of tomatoes, cherry
- 2 beaten fresh Fresh egg s, large
- 4 ounces of fat-free cheese, feta
- 25 oz. of ricotta cheese, fat-free
- 25 oz. of chopped spinach, frozen
- 1 tsp. of nutmeg, ground
- Salt, kosher
- Pepper, black, ground

Instructions:

1.

Preheat oven to 450 F.

Thaw the spinach in your microwave oven.

2. Squeeze it and drain water.

3. Mix ricotta cheese with kosher salt, ground pepper, basil, nutmeg, spinach and fresh egg s in large sized bowl. Combine well. Spray baking dish with oil. Pour in spinach mixture.

4. Spread till even. Garnish with halved cherry tomatoes. Sprinkle with cheese around tomatoes.
Place dish in oven. Cook for 45 to 50 minutes, until mixture has set well.

5. During last 6 cooking minutes, place dish under grill to brown tomatoes

and cheese. Serve warm. It can also be served cold, if you prefer.

2 4 – General Tso's Chicken

Ingredients:

- 25 ounces of bite-size cut chicken breast or thigh meat, skinless, boneless
- 1 tbsp. of wine, Shaoxing
- 2 pinch salt, kosher
- 1/2 cup of corn starch
- Non-stick spray
- 4 minced slices of ginger, peeled
- 2 minced garlic clove
- 4 or 6 de-seeded, rinsed, dried chilies, red
- 2 stalks of green onion, only the white part, cut small
- Tso sauce, bottled

Instructions:

1.

   2 . Marinate chicken meat in kosher salt and Shaoxing wine for 25 to 30 minutes.

2. Generously coat chicken with corn starch. Heat non-stick pan.

3. Fry chicken till it turns lighter brown. Remove chicken using strainer.

4. Drain off excess fat onto paper towels.

5. Heat up skillet with 5 tbsp. of non-stick spray.

6. Add chilies, ginger and garlic into skillet. Stir fry till you can easily smell the chilies' aroma.

Pour tso sauce into skillet. When it thickens and boils, add chicken.

7. Combine by stirring with sauce. Add green onions. Stir several times. Serve hot in individual dishes.

Roasted Brussels Sprouts

Ingredients:

- 5 pounds of Brussels sprouts, frozen or fresh
- 4 tbsp. of oil, olive
- 1 tsp. of salt, kosher
- 1/2 tsp. of pepper, black
- 2 tbsp. of vinegar, balsamic
- 2 tsp. of honey, organic

Instructions:

1.
   Preheat the oven to 426 F. Line large sized cookie sheet with baking paper.
   2. Trim ends from Brussels sprouts.

Peel off any wilted leaves and toss them.

2. Arrange the Brussels sprouts on cookie sheet. Use oil to drizzle. Season using kosher salt and ground pepper. Toss and coat the sprouts evenly. Spread them out into one layer with no pieces overlapping.

3. Roast the Brussels sprouts for 2 6 -25 minutes, till the edges are caramelized. Remove them from the oven.

4. Whisk vinegar and honey together in small sized bowl. Pour this mixture over the roasted Brussels sprouts. Evenly coat by tossing and serve promptly.

Sticky Asian Chicken

Ingredients:

- 8 chicken tenders or thighs, boneless, skinless
- 4 tbsp. of vinegar, balsamic
- 4 tbsp. of soy sauce, low sodium
- 2 tsp. of Splenda®
- 2 tsp. of chili paste

Instructions:

1. Brown each side of chicken pieces in skillet pre-sprayed with non-stick spray.

2. Thighs will usually take about five minutes per side, and tenders will often be done in three minutes per side.

3. Combine remainder of ingredients in sauce pan.

4. Bring to boil. Simmer for five minutes. Mixture should have thickened.

5. After chicken is browned, add sauce to skillet.

6. Cook for about five to 25 minutes for chicken thighs or five to seven minutes for chicken tenders. Serve.

Scallops in Ham Wrap

Ingredients:

- 2 lb. of scallops, large
- 4 oz. of prosciutto, sliced thinly
- 2 tbsp. of oil, olive
- 1/2 tsp. of pepper, black, ground
- 4 tbsp. of wine, white

Instructions:

1.

   Wrap the scallops in thin prosciutto slices. Secure them with toothpicks.

2. Heat oil in large sized skillet on med-high. Place scallops in pan.

3. Cook for two or three minutes per side. Season both sides with the pepper while they cook.

4. Once both sides are fried, sprinkle wine over them. Cook for one or two additional minutes.

5. Remove scallops from pan and allow to drain on plate lined with paper towels. When cooled a bit, transfer them to tray. Remove toothpicks and serve.

2 8 – Dukan Moussaka

Ingredients:

- 2 pounds of beef, ground
- 2 sliced fresh egg plants, large
- 2 onion, chopped
- 2 can of tomatoes, diced
- 2 cup of wine, red
- 2 tbsp. of oregano, dried
- Chopped parsley, fresh
- 2 tsp. of cinnamon, ground
- 2 fresh Fresh egg s, large
- 1 cup of bran, oat
- 4 tbsp. of grated Parmesan cheese
- A dash of nutmeg, ground

For the sauce

- 4   cups of milk, skim
- 2   tbsp.   of   milk
- 2 tbsp. of corn starch
- A dash of nutmeg and cinnamon
- 1/2 cup of Parmesan cheese, grated

Instructions:

1. Preheat oven to 4 6 0 degrees F.

2. Make the sauce by bringing milk almost to boil. Add corn starch. Constantly stir till consistency thickens.
    Add fresh egg yolks, cheese, nutmeg and cinnamon. Stir constantly till sauce is thick. Set aside to cool while you make the remainder.

3. Sauté beef and onion with nonstick spray.   Drain.

Add the oregano, tomatoes and wine. Simmer for 45 minutes. Place the fresh egg plant on cookie sheet.

4. Grill till browned lightly.

5. Add oat bran, fresh egg whites and cheese to the meat sauce. Remove from heat.

6. Spray cooking dish with nonstick spray.

7. Layer dish using half of fresh egg plant, all of meat mixture and then remainder of fresh egg plant.

8. Pour sauce over top. Add nutmeg and Parmesan cheese. Place in the oven. Bake for an hour.

Serve.

Dukan Tacos

Ingredients:

For taco shells

- 1/2 cup of bran, oat
- 2 fresh Fresh egg , large
- 2 scoop of protein powder, unflavored
- 1/2 tsp. of salt, kosher
- 1/2 tsp. of pepper, ground
- 1 tsp. of garlic powder
- 1 tsp. of onion powder
- 1 cup of cheddar cheese shreds, fat free
- 2 to 2 tbsp. of water, filtered

For the beef

• 2 pound of ground beef, extra lean
• 2   pkt. of seasoning mix, taco
• 1/2 cup of water, filtered
• To serve: cheddar cheese shreds, fat free

Instructions:

To   create   taco   shells
Blend all ingredients outside of water in
food   processor.
Add 2 -2 tbsp. of water to create your
desired   consistency.
Preheat a pan with non-stick spray over
med-high.

Pour 1/2 of batter after another into
pan. Tilt and form a five to six-inch
tortilla.
Cook for two or three minutes till edge

forms a crust. Flip. Cook for one to two more minutes.

 To prepare meat and assemble the tacos Brown beef lightly in large size pan. Add taco seasoning and 1/2 cup of water. Stir and bring to boil. Reduce to simmer and simmer for five minutes.

Serve seasoned beef and chosen condiments on homemade tortillas.

Basil Thai Chicken

Ingredients:

- Non-stick spray
- 4 minced garlic cloves
- 2 to 6 chopped, pounded bird (Thai) chilies
- 2 diced shallots
- 1 pound of cubed chicken, boneless
- 2 tbsp. of fish sauce, Thai
- 2-4 tsp. of soy sauce, sweet, black, as desired
- 2 tsp. of Splenda®
- 2 pinch pepper, WHITE
- Large bunch stem-removed Thai basil, sweet
- 2 fresh Fresh egg s, large
- Optional: 2 slivered lime leaves, kaffir

Instructions:

Spray heated skillet, then add shallots and garlic. Stir fry them till they are aromatic.

Add chicken meat. Stir fry quickly. Break chicken meat into small sized lumps.

When chicken has changed color, add chilies and seasonings. Continue stir-frying.

Add basil leaves. Stir a few times till basil leaves wilt and you smell their exotic fragrance.

Sprinkle 2 dashes of white pepper powder in mixture. Stir one last time. Transfer to dishes. Serve promptly.

Zucchini Cheese Roll-ups

Ingredients:

• 4 or 4 zucchinis, large, sliced in 2 /4"
pieces
•   Spreadable   cheese,   light
•   Spinach   leaves,   baby
•   Salt,   kosher
•   Pepper,   ground   black
• Oil, olive

Instructions:

Spray the zucchini with oil. Season them
with kosher salt ground pepper. Grill till
tender.

At one edge of zucchini, place 1 to 2 tsp.
cheese mixture and spinach. Roll them

up and serve them with the seam facing down.

22 – Dukan Fresh egg Noodles

Ingredients:

- 2 fresh Fresh egg s, large
- 5 tbsp. of corn meal
- Salt, kosher
- Pepper, black, ground

Instructions:

Crack fresh egg s into bowl and add kosher salt and ground pepper. Mix fresh egg s till batter is smooth.. Add the corn meal. Use a spoon to pour the batter into boiling broth. Don't stir it. Turn heat off when all batter is in broth and it has begun to boil again. Serve noodles   hot.

Portobello Crust Pizza

Ingredients:

- 6 de-stemmed large mushrooms, Portobello
- 2 tbsp. of oil, olive
- 2 lb. of Italian sausage, mild
- 2 x 2 6 -oz. can of pizza sauce
- 2 chopped green pepper, medium
- 2 chopped onion, medium
- 1 cup of chopped mushrooms, fresh
- 1/2 cup of grated cheese, Parmesan
- 2 minced cloves of garlic
- 2 cup of mozzarella cheese shreds,

part-skim
• Optional: basil leaves, sliced

Instructions:

1.

Place the mushrooms with the stem facing down on pregreased cookie sheet and drizzle them with oil. 2. Bake for 25 to 26 minutes at 4 6 0F till tender. Turn them once.

2. Cook sausage on med. heat till it shows no pink. Drain it. Add and stir pizza sauce, garlic, Parmesan cheese, mushrooms, onion and pepper. Divide sauce among the mushrooms and sprinkle them with mozzarella cheese.

3. Broil two to three inches from heat for one to two minutes till cheese

melts. Sprinkle with fresh basil, as desired. Serve.

Dukan Deviled Fresh egg s

Ingredients:

- 4 fresh Fresh egg s, large
- 5 tbsp. of nonfat mayonnaise
- 2 tsp. of mustard, Dijon
- As desired: paprika, kosher salt, ground pepper

Instructions:

Cover the fresh egg s with water in pot on stove. Place on high heat. Bring the water to boil. Cover hot and turn heat off. Leave the fresh egg s covered for about 2 0-30 minutes.

Remove the pot from stove top. Drain hot water off. Run fresh egg s under cold water till they are cooled. Once cooled, peel and slice them lengthways. Spoon yolks into separate bowl.

Mash the yolks together with mayo, along with kosher salt, ground pepper and mustard till consistency is smooth. Spoon filling evenly among fresh egg white halves. Sprinkle over using paprika and serve them cold.

Crust Vegetable Quiche

Ingredients:

- 2 small yellow squash, sliced
- 2 small zucchinis, sliced
- 2 chopped bell pepper, orange
- 2 chopped, roasted garlic cloves
- 2 tbsp. of thyme, ground
- 4 fresh Fresh egg s, large
- 4 fresh egg whites, large
- 1/3 cup of milk, 2%
- 1/3 tsp. of salt, kosher
- 1/2 tsp. of pepper, black ground
- 1/2 cup of cheese, shredded
- 2 tbsp. of Parmesan cheese, grated

Instructions:

1.

   Heat large sized skillet on med-high. Spray with the nonstick spray. Add zucchini, squash, pepper, thyme and garlic.

2. Cook for six to seven minutes and stir frequently, till vegetables are all tender. Spoon them into a medium sized bowl. Let them cool while you work on fresh egg mixture.

3. Preheat the oven to 4 6 0 degrees F. Spray 10 " square pan using non-stick spray. Set it aside. Whisk fresh Fresh egg s, milk, fresh egg whites, milk, kosher salt and ground pepper together in large sized bowl till combined well.

4. Arrange the vegetables into prepped pan. Top them with the shredded cheese. Top that with fresh egg mixture. Sprinkle with Parmesan cheese.

5. Place pan in oven. Bake for 40-50 minutes till filling has set and doesn't jiggle anymore. Cool for 8-25 minutes on wire rack. Slice and serve.

Spiced Rhubarb Compote and Orange Cream

Ingredients:

- 2 1/3 oz. of peeled, grated ginger
- 4 tbsp. of sweetener, your choice
- 25 1 ounces of trimmed, cubed rhubarb

- 4   tbsp. of yogurt, Greek, fat-free
- 4   tbsp. of crème fraiche, low-fat
- 2 orange, zest only, grated

Instructions:

1. Place sweetener and ginger in pan with 6 fluid oz. of filtered water. Bring to boil. Simmer for two or three minutes.

2. Stir in rhubarb. Simmer for four to five minutes. Remove from heat. Cover pan and allow to cool. Stir now and   then. Beat orange zest, yogurt and crème fraiche together. Serve rhubarb compote under a dollop of the orange cream.

Oat Bran Cookies

Ingredients:

- 1/3 cup of bran, oat
- 1/2 tsp. of baking soda
- 2 /8 tsp. of salt, kosher
- 2 tbsp. of Splenda® brown sugar substitute
- 2 pkts. of regular Splenda®
- 2 tbsp. of milk, skim
- Nonstick spray

Instructions:

Preheat the oven to 4 8 6 F. Blend oat bran, Splenda®, brown sugar Splenda®, salt and baking soda in food processor.

Pour the mixture in medium bowl. Add milk. Spray nonstick spray into the mixture for a second. Combine ingredients well.

Form six cookies. Place them on baking paper. Bake for 6 -8 minutes. Remove from   oven   and   serve.

Vanilla Meringue Cookies

Ingredients:

- 4 room-temperature fresh egg whites from large fresh egg s
- 1/2 tsp. of cream o' tartar
- 8 tbsp. of Splenda® sweetener, granulated
- 1/3 tsp. of vanilla extract, pure

Instructions:

1.

Preheat the oven to 26 0F. Line baking sheets using parchment paper.

2. Beat the fresh egg whites till foamy. Add cream o' tartar. Beat on high till it forms soft peaks. Add sweetener in gradually as you beat.

3. Continue beating on high speed till peaks are quite stiff. Add vanilla extract. Mix till combined well.

   Put meringue in piping bag. Pipe dollops on cookie sheets. Bake for an hour and 10 minutes. Allow them to cool in turned off, closed oven. Remove carefully from the oven. Serve or place in airtight container. Refrigerate leftover cookies.

Oat Bran Vanilla-Orange Muffins

Ingredients:

- 8 tbsp. of bran, oat
- 1 cup of fresh egg whites, large
- 6 tbsp. of orange yogurt, non-fat
- 2 tsp. of baking powder
- 2 tsp. of Splenda® sweetener
- 2 tbsp. of vanilla pudding powder, sugar free
- 2 tsp. of orange extract, pure

Instructions:

Mix dry ingredients in large bowl. Add fresh egg s and yogurt. Whisk till smooth. Add the extract. Evenly divide mixture in 2 2 mini muffin tins pre-sprayed using oil. Bake in 4 6 0F oven for 2 2 -30 minutes. Remove from oven and serve.

Berries Meringue

Ingredients:

- 2 cup each of blueberries, strawberries and raspberries
- 2 tbsp. of honey, organic
- For meringue
- 6 fresh egg whites from large fresh eggs
- 2 tbsp. of sugar substitute, granulated
- Optional: 1 tsp. of xanthan gum
- 2 tsp. of vinegar, white

Instructions:

1. Wash, then slice berries. Combine with sweetener in medium sized bowl.

2. Toss gently to coat the berries. Spoon into six small-sized baking dishes.

91

3. For meringue

4. Combine xanthan gum, fresh egg whites and sweetener in large sized bowl. Whip till it forms stiff peaks. Add vinegar. Whip till barely combined.

5. Spoon meringue over berries.

6. Bake in 4 00F oven for 20-26 minutes for the six small sized meringues.
Remove. Serve promptly.

Sautéed White Fish in Red Sauce

Ingredients:

i¼   tsp.   chili   powder

2   tbsp. fresh cilantro, chopped

2   garlic   cloves,   crushed

1   tsp,   ground   cumin

4   tbsp.   fresh lemon juice

Zest   of   2   lemon

2   small onion, sliced finely

2   tbsp. fresh parsley, chopped

2   red pepper, finely sliced

2   tsp.   sweet   paprika

8   oz canned tomato, chopped

1   tsp.   turmeric

2   4   oz   firm   white   fish

Directions

1.

Mix all marinade ingredients together in bowl.

2. Place fish in a single layer inside a casserole dish, and sprinkle evenly with marinade.

3. Allow to marinate at least 2 hours. coat the fish in the marinade.

4. Leave to marinade for a minimum of 2   hours,   or   overnight.

Preheat oven to 4 6 0°F.

Sauté onion in a non-stick frying pan until tender.

5. Add garlic, fresh lemon zest and spices. Cook for 2 minutes.

6. Add garlic, fresh lemon zest and spices and cook for 2 minutes.

7. Add red pepper and chopped canned tomatoes. Bring mixture to a simmer, and cook gently for 10 minutes.

8. Salt and pepper to taste. Spread the sauce evenly over the fish and bake in the oven for 25 minutes, or until the fish cab be flaked with a fork.

Lightly Sweetened Chocolate Wedges

Ingredients

2 fresh egg

6 tbsp. oat bran

2 tbsp. sweetener

6 tbsp. low-fat vanilla yogurt 2 tsp. baking powder

2 tbsp. low-fat, unsweetened cocoa powder

Directions

1.

Preheat oven to 4 6 0°F.
Put all ingredients into a medium
sized bowl, and mix well.

2. Place batter into parchment-lined 6"
round baking tin.

3. Bake for 25-30 minutes, and remove
while still soft in the center. Allow to
cool for a few minutes and cut into 6
wedges.

Tofu and fresh egg ie Stir-Fry

Ingredients

Juice from 2 lemon

2 tsp. lemongrass, crushed

8 oz. firm tofu, cut into even-sized pieces

2 tbsp. low-sodium soy sauce

1 c. broccoli florets

2 zucchini, sliced

2 garlic clove, finely chopped

2 tsp. fresh ginger, grated

Directions

1.

Mix the garlic, ginger, lemongrass, fresh lemon juice and soy sauce together in a bowl.

2. Add tofu to a non-stick frying pan on a high heat.

3. Stir often to prevent the tofu sticking. Once the tofu is lightly browned, add vegetables and 2 tablespoons of water.

4. Stir contents of skillet for a few minutes until they are cooked, but still quite firm.

5. Add soy sauce, and cook for another minute.

Chilled Seafood Salad

Ingredients:

4 lemons

Fresh parsley (to taste)

2 lb scallops

2 lb shrimp, cleaned and de-veined 2 lb calamari, cut into bite size pieces

2 celery stalks, diced

2-4 garlic cloves, finely chopped or pressed

Directions:

1.

Set a large pot of water to boil.

2. Cut up a half of lemon, and squeeze fresh juice into boiling water.

3. Also throw in juiced lemon. Boil shrimp for approximately 6 minutes (until pink). Remove with slotted spoon and set in an ice bath.

4. When cool, cut into bite-sized pieces. Then, add calamari to boil. Cook for about 4 minutes (until opaque). Remove with slotted spoon and set aside to cool.

5. Add scallops to same pot. Cook for 10 minutes.

6. Set aside to cool. In a large container (with lid), place garlic, celery, juice of

2 lemons, cooled seafood, parsley, salt and pepper.

7. Cover container and shake well. Refrigerate for at least 2 hours before serving.

Italian Sausage and Noodles in Cream Sauce

Ingredients

2 c. fat-free milk

Fresh parsley (to taste)

Tofu Shirataki Noodles

2 pack chicken sausage (spicy Italian), about 6 links

2 oz fat-free cream cheese

Directions

1.

Remove the sausage from casing, and brown in a non-stick skillet over medium heat.

2. Once cooked, add milk and cream cheese. Bring to a low boil and reduce heat.

3. Prepare noodles according to package directions.

4. Add cooked noodles to sausage mixture.

5. Cook a bit more until noodles well coated and sauce thickens.

6. Garnish with parsley.

Fromage Frais Gateau

Ingredients

• Vz tsp sweetener

• 2 fresh egg yolks

• 4 fresh egg whites

• 4 drops of oil

• 250g (4 1 oz) virtually fat-free fromage frais

•50g (2 oz) cornflour

• 2 tsp yeast

• Grated zest of 2 fresh lemon

Instructions

1. 2 . Preheat the oven to 200c/400f/gas 6. Mix together ingredients, bar the fresh egg whites and oil.
2. Fold the stiffly beaten fresh egg whites into this mixture.
3. Pour into oiled cake tin, cook for 45 minutes. Serve
4. chilled.

Meatballs With Rosemary

Ingredients

- 2 tbsp Chinese plum sauce

- 2 tbsp Worcestershire sauce

- 2 tbsp rosemary, finely chopped

- 2 -2 tbsp mint or basil, finely chopped

- Salt and black pepper

- 2 medium onion, chopped

- 900g (lib lOoz) minced beef

- 2 garlic cloves, crushed

- 2 fresh egg, lightly beaten

Instructions

1. Mix together all the ingredient and then shape into
2. meatballs the size of a walnut.
3. Cook the meatballs, a few at a time, in a saucepan over a medium heat for about five minutes until they
4. are golden-brown on all sides.
5. Allow any fat to drain off on to kitchen paper.

Veggie Curry

Ingredients

- 2 fresh onion chopped half an aubergine

- 2 gloves of garlic bunch of spinach

- 2 fresh eggs

- uorn chicken pieces

- 25 cherry tomatoes or 6 large tomatoes cut into uarters half a large butternut suash cut into cubes

- 20g of pataks tikka masala paste non DD but only

6 2kcal/4 g carb/4g fat

Instructions

1. Sweat the onions & garlic in a wok.
2. Marinate the chicken in the paste, add to wok.
3. Add tomatoes & aubergine, add half a cup of water, add the part boiled suash and 2 hard boiled fresh eggs cut into uarters, leave to simmer for 25 minutes, add in spinach.

Mussel Ceviche

Ingredients

• 2 Cloves Garlic

• 1 a Cucumber

• 1 a Jalapeno

• Salt, Pepper, Dried Basil

• Mussels (De-shelled package from the Asian market)

• 1 a Red Onion

• 1 a Fresh lemon

• Cilantro

• 2 Tomatoes

Instructions

2 . Saute mussels until cooked through. Set aside to cool.

2. Cut all ingredients into diced pieces.

4 . Season with salt, pepper, dried basil and any other spices you like.

4. Sueeze some fresh fresh lemon juice and mix ingredients well.

6 . Chill for a bit and serve.

Pizza Stuffed Peppers

Ingredients

- 2 green pepper

- Cooked Ground Italian Turkey Sausage

- Turkey Pepperoni

- 2 Tomato, pureed

- Cooked, diced fresh onion

- Cooked, minced garlic

- Oregano to taste

- FF mozzarella (or low fat feta is really good too) Instructions

2 . Preheat oven to 4 6 0 degrees.

2. Fill bottom of pepper with cooked turkey sausage.

4 . Mix tomato, onion, garlic and oregano.

4. Top sausage with 1 tomato mixutre.

6 . Add pepperoni.

6. Top with tomato mixture and sprinkle with mozzarella

cheese. Place stuffed pepper on baking sheet and bake

uncovered for 45 minutes.

8 . Sausage and pepperoni can be replaced with lean ground beef and/or cooked turkey bacon.

Dukan Micro Bread With Marmite

Ingredients

- 2 fresh egg

- tablespoon uark,

- 0.6 teaspoon baking powder,

- 2 Tablespoon Oat bran,

- 2 tablespoon wheat bran,

Instructions

1. Mix up with a fork put into a shallow 4" suare micro
2. dish, cook for 4 minutes in the microwave, let it rest for a minute then slice thinly i got 4 nice slices, and i could eat them without toasting them, i ate them straight away lovely and warm from the oven,mix 2 tablespoon
3. Quark with 1 teaspoon marmite until it was well blended together, oh boy! it did the job, delicious, this
4. is definetely going to be a regular favourite, comfort food at its best

Pseudo Jambalaya

Ingredients

- 2   chicken breast, cooked Tobasco sauce to taste

- 2 T minced Garlic

- 2 half small onion, diced

- Freshly ground pepper

- 2   package Shirataki Angel Hair Noodles, drained, cut to rice length

- 1 package Turkey Kielbasa, cut into chunks

Instructions

1. Stir fry (in water, or in pan sprayed with fat free
2. cooking spray) garlic, onion, cooked chicken breast, and kielbasa. (Add other vegies at this point if desired.) 2 06
3. Add shirataki to pan and stir fry until noodles start to
4. shrink (this changes the texture so they aren't so
5. suishy).
6. Add Tobasco to taste

Baked Eggs In Ham Cups

Ingredients

• Vegetables of choice (If PV)

• Salt, pepper and other seasonings as desired Instructions

• 2 fresh egg

• 2 thinly sliced piece of 10 8 % ham or turkey ham

• FF cheese of choice (I use ff Cheddar)

2 . Preheat oven to 400 degrees F.

2. Line a small ramekin or muffin pan with the piece of ham. Fill with cheese and vegetables (if applicable) and top with egg.

4 . Bake in oven for about 25 minutes or until the fresh egg white is hard but the yolk is still soft.

4. To serve, remove from ramekin and serve on a plate

Oriental Salmon With Sweet Soy And Ginger Sauce

Ingredients:

• pinch of pepper

• grated ginger

• chopped coriander leaves

• 2 sliced chilli (if you like it spicy)

• Salmon fillets (as much as you like)

• 4 tbsp soy sauce

• 2 tbsp splenda/other sweetener

Instructions

1. 2 . Preheat oven to 2 80C
2. Mix soy sauce, splenda and pepper to form the sweet soy sauce.
3. 4 . Place salmon fillets on a big piece of foil. Spoon the
4. sauce all over the fillets on both sides, saving ltbsp for later.
5. Sprinkle the ginger, coriander and chilli on top of the
6. salmon then pour the remaining sauce over this.
7. 6 . Gather the edges of the foil and scrunch the edges
8. together to form a closed packet.
9. Place in baking tray in the oven and cook for 25 mins.

Turkey And Vegetable Chili

Ingredients

• 2 Clove Garlic

• Sour Cream to Garnish

• 2 Can of Pickled Jalapenos and Carrots

• Mixture of Cumin, Cinnamon, Red Chili Pepper, Salt, Pepper

• 2 Green Onion

• 3 lbs of Ground Turkey

• 1 to 2 Red Onion

• 260 oz Can of Tomato Sauce

• 250oz Can of Diced Tomatoes

Instructions

1. Saute ground turkey.
2. While turkey is cooking, dice up your onion, garlic, jalapenos and carrots. Prepare spice mixture.
3. Drain the turkey fat and add your spice mixture. Add some reserved liuid (about 1/2 cup) from the diced tomatoes. Cook for 4 minutes.
4. Add the onions, jalapenos and carrots and cook for 6
5. minutes.
6. Lastly, add the diced tomatoes and tomato sauce.
7. Simmer for 45 minutes or until sauce has thickened a bit.
8. Serve with a dollop of fat free sour cream and garnish with green onion

Asian Beef

Ingredients

• Sliced red pepper, mushrooms, onions

• Bok Choy cabbage

• Pour over 1/2 cup beef stock

• 2 Tbsp Soy sauce

• Beef Steak - into strips and fry off with:

• 4 TSP fresh ginger.

• 2 garlic cloves

Instructions

1. Simmer and cook through to get the full flavours

Dill Salmon With Cauliflower Puree

Ingredients for Salmon

• Salmon

• Fresh Dill

• Half a Lemon

• Salt, Pepper, Onion Powder

Ingredients for Cauliflower Puree

- Cauliflower

- Skimmed Milk

- Non-Fat Sour Cream

- Garlic

Instructions

1. Sueeze some fresh lemon juice (half a lemon) on the
2. salmon and sprinkle salt, pepper and onion powder on it. For this recipe, I used fresh dill, placing a bed of dill for the salmon to rest on as well on top.
3. Place it in the broiler until salmon becomes slightly
4. opaue (approximately 25 minutes).
5. For the cauliflower puree, boil two cups worth until just tender.
6. Place in blender with some

7. reserved liuid, salt, pepper, a little garlic, a dash of skimmed milk and non-fat sour cream. Blend until you are happy with the consistency.
8. Plate and garnish with some more fresh dill.

Vietnamese Beef

2 big piece ginger, grated

4 drops vegetable oil

4 garlic cloves, crushed

400g sirloin steak, cut into 2 cm cubes

2 tbs soy sauce

2 tbs oyster sauce

Coriander leaves, to serve

1. Combine beef, sauces, ginger and a little black pepper.
2. Marinate for at least 45 minutes. Brown garlic in a pan
3. Add beef and stir over high heat for 25-30 seconds for medium-rare. Top with coriander.

Oat Bran Pancake

- 290 g flaked tuna, smoked salmon, ham or chicken
- 2 eggs, separated
- Oil, for cooking
- 5 tbs oat bran
- 5 tbs fat-free quark
- Dried herbs, optional

1. Stir oat bran into quark with herbs, a pinch of salt and pepper, fish, meat or chicken and fresh egg yolks.
2. Beat eggwhites until stiff peaks form, then fold into oat bran mixture.
3. Pour into a non-stick pan that has been oiled and wiped with kitchen paper and a few drops of oil.
4. Cook for 5-10 minutes each side.

Baked Fish With Herbs

6 tbs chopped herbs

4 drops vegetable oil

800g white fish fillets

4 00g fat-free fromage frais

4 fresh eggs

1. Preheat oven to 220ºC. Season fish fillets and wrap in greaseproof paper.
2. Bake for 25 minutes. Reduce heat to 2 80ºC. Remove fish from oven.
3. Put cooked fillets into a blender with fromage frais, fresh eggs and herbs and blend well.
4. Pour mixture into a baking dish

139

5. Place dish into a bigger dish. Half fill bigger dish with cold water. Bake for 50 minutes or until cooked through.

Fresh Lemon Cheesecake

4 00g fat-free cream cheese

2 tbsp cornflour

8 tbsp sweetener

2 fresh eggs

4 tbsp fromage frais

4 tbsp uark

200g cottage cheese

grated lemon zest

1. Heat oven to 2 60ºC. Mix ingredients except fresh egg whites and cornflour and beat until smooth and thick. In another bowl, beat the fresh egg whites until stiff, then add the cornflour.
2. Fold this mixture into the first bowl. in a dish, bake for 45 minutes or until risen and golden brown. Cool, then serve garnished with grated lemon zest.

Lunch: Rosemary Beef Burgers

900g minced beef

2 onion, chopped

2 garlic cloves, crushed

2 tbs plum sauce

2 tbs Worcestershire sauce

2 tbs finely chopped rosemary

2 -2 tbs finely chopped mint or basil

2 fresh egg, lightly beaten

Salad to serve, optional

1. Combine all ingredients, season with salt and pepper to taste and shape into patties.
2. Grill until golden brown on both sides and cooked through. Drain on paper towel.

Fishcake

2 garlic clove, crushed

Chopped herbs, to taste

2 white fish fillet, chopped

4 crabsticks, thinly sliced

4 eggs, separated

6 tbs fat-free uark

2 tbs cornflour

1. Beat eggwhites until stiff. Add other ingredients and bake in a lined tin at 2 80ºC for 410 minutes.

Chocolate Coffee Meringues

6 tbsp sweetener

2 tsp very strong coffee

4 fresh egg whites

2 tsp cocoa powder

1. Preheat the oven to 2 6 0ºC. Beat the fresh egg whites until very stiff.
2. Add the cocoa to the sweetener, then sprinkle this over the egg whites.

3. Add the coffee and continue beating for about 45 seconds.
4. Spoon into small mounds on a baking tray and bake for 30 to 45 minutes.

Oat Bran Muffins

4 tbs fromage frais

1 tsp sweetener

Fresh lemon zest or cinnamon

4 eggs, separated

8 tbs oat bran

1. Heat oven to 2 80ºC. Beat eggwhites until stiff.
2. Mix other ingredients. Fold in eggwhites. Pour into cases. Bake for 20-45 minutes.

Prawn And Fresh Egg Salad

A few sprigs tarragon

200g prawns, cooked and shelled

4 fresh eggs

2 tsp olive oil

4 tsp cider vinegar

650g lettuce

1. Make a vinaigrette with oil and vinegar and some salt and pepper.
2. Mix lettuce, tarragon leaves and prawns in a bowl.
3. Soft-boil eggs for 6 -6 minutes. Shell carefully as yolks will still be runny.

4. Serve eggs, while still very hot, on top of dressed lettuce and prawns.

Salmon Escalopes And Mustard Dill Sauce

6 tsp fat-free fromage frais

Finely chopped dill, to taste

Steamed asparagus,optional

4 thick (about 200g each)

pieces salmon

2 shallots, chopped

2 tbs mild mustard

1. Put salmon in the freezer for a few minutes so you can cut it into thin (about 6 0g) slices.
2. Gently fry slices in a non-stick pan for 2 minute each side.
3. Set aside and keep warm. Brown shallots. Reduce heat.
4. Add mustard and fromage frais. Simmer for 10 minutes. Return salmon to pan. Add dill. Season. Cook until heated through. Serve with asparagus.

Chocolate Pannacotta

2 tbsp protein powder

2 00ml skimmed milk

6 tbsp fat-free fromage frais

2 gelatine leaves

2 egg yolks

2 tbsp of cocoa powder

1. Place the gelatine in a bowl of cold water to soften. In another bowl, combine the fresh egg yolks, cocoa powder and protein powder, set aside.

2. Bring the milk to the boil in a small saucepan, gently pour over the fresh egg mixture and stir to combine.

3. Sueeze out any excess water from the gelatine and drop into the hot mixture,
4. then stir until fully dissolved. Allow to cool, then add the fromage frais.

Muesli And Skim Milk

2 tbs liuid sweetener

Almond essence

6 tbs oat bran

2 fresh egg

1. Preheat oven to 2 60ºC. Mix all ingredients and spread on tray lined with baking paper.
2. Bake for 45 minutes.
3. Crumble when cool. Store in an air-tight container.

Lunch: Salmon Pancakes

2 small jar salmon roe

4 slices smoked salmon

2 oat bran pancakes

4 00g fat-free fromage frais

60g fat-free quark

1. Mix fromage frais, uark and roe in a bowl. Season.
2. Divide mixture among pancakes. Top with salmon.

Chicken Kebabs

2 tbs fresh lemon juice

2 00g fat-free plain yoghurt

1 tbs ground coriander

1 tbs ground cumin

2 tsp garam masala

2 onion, peeled

2 garlic clove, peeled

20g ginger, grated

2 tbs finely chopped coriander

800g chicken breasts, cut into 2cm chunks

Fat-free tzatziki, to serve

1. Purée onion and garlic in a blender. Stir in ginger, lemon juice, yoghurt, spices and coriander.
2. Mix chicken and marinade in a bowl. Refrigerate for 2 hours. Heat a grill on high.
3. Thread chicken on skewers. Cook for 8-25 minutes. Serve with fat-free tzatziki.

Orange Yogurt Cake

2 tsp orange extract

4 tbsp cornflour

2 tsp yeast

4 drops of vegetable oil

4 fresh eggs

280g fat-free natural yogurt

1 tsp artificial sweetener

    1.   Preheat the oven to 2 80ºC. Beat fresh eggs with yogurt, then add sweetener, orange extract, corn flour and yeast. Pour into a cake tin (oiled and lined with kitchen paper) and bake for 410 minutes.

Lightning Source UK Ltd.
Milton Keynes UK
UKHW051924270522
403653UK00009B/128